# Bone Spurs explained.

## Bone Spurs Symptoms, Causes, Exercises and Treatments all covered.

## Includes Neck, Foot, Heel, Shoulder, Spine, Knee, Cervical, Hip Joint, Hand and Wrist bone spurs.

by

**Robert Rymore**

Published by IMB Publishing 2013

# Table of Contents

# Preface

Ageing is a natural phenomenon that none of us can escape. With advancing age come changes in almost every part of our body – our skin, our eyesight, our organs and even our joints. Osteoarthritis is a clinical condition that affects over millions of people all over the world. Bone spurs are a feature of osteoarthritis and can also be seen as a consequence of a number of other clinical conditions too.

Bone spurs can occur in the presence of a number of risk factors. In this e-book, we have taken a detailed look into the common risk factors, particularly integrating these risks into management strategies that can help treat or even prevent bone spurs. As a patient who suffers from bone spurs, it is worthwhile having a good knowledge of how these bone spurs develop, which in turn will help you as a patient to identify factors in your life that may be contributing to their development. After all, knowledge is power!

We have also taken a close look at the normal anatomy of various joints and structures within the joint where bone spurs can develop. The symptoms and signs patients can experience have also been discussed. While the primary symptom of bone spurs is pain, it may come as a surprise that bone spurs can also cause nerve compression and muscle weakness, especially when they are located in the spine. When located in the hand, they can cause difficulty in small movements of the hand that can impact a patient's life significantly. In fact, some patients may find it difficult to hold their morning cup of tea or even write. The impact can really be that severe.

We have attempted to provide a few simple measures at home that will help manage the pain and allow for increased mobility when it comes to performing simple tasks. However, these measures unfortunately do not offer a cure. The problem with bone spurs is the notoriety in returning once they have been treated. It is for this reason that most patients who suffer from bone spurs are offered symptom control alone. In patients in whom the pain is unbearable and quality of life is affected to a point where they cannot perform simple household tasks, surgery may be offered. This of course has risks, and we have covered this aspect briefly as well. Remember to always discuss any procedure in detail before you undergo any surgical treatments with your doctor.

Finally, we would like to thank you for reading this book. We hope that the information enclosed is useful and beneficial in understanding this rather troublesome illness. We would like to kindly remind you that all the material in this e-book is meant for information purposes only, and we strongly recommend that you seek the advice of a doctor before embarking on any treatment. Remember that symptoms due to bone spurs can be treated easily.

We hope you enjoy reading this e-book as much as we have enjoyed writing it!

# Chapter 1 - Introduction

At some point in our lives, we have all suffered from some form of pain. This pain may be in our shoulders, back, neck or even feet. There can be a number of causes of pain in people, and many a time it is due to a sprained or strained muscle or tendon due to our very own sheer clumsiness. In some cases, it can be due to a bone spur.

The human body is made up of 206 bones in total. This includes the 33 bones in our spine, the bones in our hips, shoulders and the tiny bones in the hands and feet. As we grow and get older, our bones are subject to a lot of wear and tear from all the different activities we perform and the stresses we place them under. It is no surprise therefore that some form of arthritis can occur in sites where there is most wear and tear. It is at these sites that sometimes bone spurs can occur.

A bone spur refers to a projection of bone that grows from a bone that already exists – a 'bony outgrowth', so to speak. In the medical world, it is called an 'osteophyte'. Formally known as interior ankle impingement syndrome, bone spurs are common among athletes and people who engage in high impact activities such as running. Developing a bone spur is not a common occurrence and it can be quite annoying to patients. The reason for this is that the bone spurs can compress on nearby structures and this is what causes the pain. The bone spurs by themselves are not painful. Depending on its location, bone spurs can have an impact on movement and can therefore directly affect a patient's quality of life.

In this book, we shall take a closer look at why bone spurs develop, what the causes are, types of bone spurs, clinical features and the treatment of this condition in various cases.

# Chapter 2 – Definition and Patho-physiology

## 1. Definition – The 'What'

In the previous chapter, we took a very brief look at what bone spurs are. In essence, and by definition, bone spurs or 'osteophytes' are projections of bone from existing bone. The latter fact is important to remember, as sometimes tiny spurs can grow from joint tissues and tendons called enthesophytes. These are completely different from bone spurs.

Unlike what the name would suggest, 'spur' does not refer to the projection being sharp and pointy. Instead, bone spurs bear the characteristic feature of being rather smooth. By themselves, bone spurs are painless. The pain that patients do experience with bone spurs occurs due to the spur impinging on or placing pressure upon a nerve or any other structure nearby. For example, a spur of the calcaneum (heel bone) can place undue pressure on the heel when walking, causing difficulty to the patient when they walk or even stand for a while in one place. There is no doubt that this can be distressing and annoying, and can prompt patients to seek treatment just so that they can regain their quality of life and mobility back again.

That was just one example of a bone spur. In subsequent chapters we shall take a look at the different sites at which that bone spurs occur and what symptoms they cause.

Now that you have a basic understanding of what bone spurs refer to, let us take a look at the all-important question that doctors and physical therapists get asked all the time – ' How do bone spurs develop?'

## 2. Patho-physiology – The 'How'

When we move our bodies, different parts of them work in perfect synchrony to allow for smooth movement. This movement requires the use of muscles, joints, tendons and even the bones to work together. It is only natural that, with years and years of movement, the bones and joints in our body are placed under a variety of stresses. For example, take a look at weight lifters. By lifting heavy weights, they are placing their shoulders and their backs under a lot of stress. With years of weight lifting and constant training, there is no doubt that their bones and joints can become damaged.

### a. The role of stress and inflammation

In some patients, these years of stress and wear and tear can result in a condition called osteoarthritis. Literally defined, osteoarthritis refers to inflammation of the bones and joints, though from a scientific point of view it refers to damage to the cartilage that surrounds the bone. Bear in mind that osteoarthritis is usually seen in older individuals. However, in people who enjoy sports, the constant strain can lead to some damage over a shorter period of time, resulting in osteoarthritis occurring a lot sooner. In some cases, there may be a medical reason why these changes can occur in younger individuals.

Under all this damage and stress, small parts of the bone are worn off. This can result in inflammation of the affected area, which triggers the body to make an attempt to replace this bone by forming new bone in the area. However, the problem that can arise is that instead of the new bone just filling out the area that has now been eroded, the growth overfills and outgrows the space. This is the bone spur. It usually is quite a smooth growth and not a sharp one.

Let's take a look at another example – the spine. Our spine supports our body. It maintains an upright posture and pretty much bears the entire weight of the body when it does so. The formation of bone spurs in the vertebrae (bones of the back) is a natural phenomenon that occurs with ageing. It indicates that the bones and tissues in the spine are getting worn out and old, and that in order to maintain its health it is growing new bone. Bone spurs can occur anywhere along the spine, and by themselves do not cause any problems. In fact, bone spurs may not even be diagnosed in patients until they have an x-ray or they develop some sort of pain. The pain that does occur is because these bone spurs are in a place they should not be; and they are compressing the nerves that arise from the spinal cord. As these nerves supply the various parts of the body, it is natural that pain or tingling sensations occur in the parts of the body that are supplied by these nerves.

## b. Contribution from sports and athletics

In patients who enjoy sports and other outdoor activities, injuries are common. When a joint injury occurs, there is damage to the structures within that joint, which includes the joint cartilage and the bone. Resting the joint is the best way to allow the injured structure to heal. When resting, the body tries to rebuild the tissue that has been damaged due to the injury. This usually occurs rather smoothly and without a fault. However, if the patient suffers repeated injury at the same site over and over again, then the healing of the tissue can alter, and bone spurs can develop at the site. For example, athletes and footballers are constantly on their feet, subjecting them to constant pounding on the ground and different kinds of stretches and movements during kicking and jumping. This can place a great deal of stress on the ankle joint, particularly because many of the movements are not natural. Eventually, bone spurs can develop around the ankles that can place pressure on the tissues that encase the front of the ankle joint. This is called anterior (front) ankle impingement, and can be a bothersome condition for sportspersons.

In a nutshell, the pathophysiology of bone spurs can be described in 3 steps –

Step – 1: Ageing of the joint structures (osteoarthritis) or constant injury to the bones and joints that encompasses years.

Step – 2: Bone growth at the site of injury or stress in an attempt to fill the area that has been damaged. Constant injury only stimulates more bone growth, resulting in bone spurs being formed.

Step – 3: Pressure of the bone spurs on surrounding structures like the nerves and muscles, causing pain and discomfort. In some cases, patients may not experience any symptoms whatsoever.

## Chapter 3 – Prevalence of Bone Spurs – How Common Are They?

If one were to look at bone spurs, they would no doubt agree from our previous discussion that bone spurs are seen more often in athletes and people who use their joints a lot more than they should. While this remains a fact, it does not provide a good idea about how common bone spurs actually are.

### a. Why is it important to know?

Estimating how common a condition is in the general public is called 'prevalence' of that condition. From a statistical point of view, it is good to know how big a clinical condition is amongst people as it gives the treating physician a good idea as to how to investigate and manage it effectively. Furthermore, analysing the prevalence on a regular basis allows public health authorities to realise whether the problem is a rapidly growing one, and what sort of resources need to be allocated to treat the condition.

In the medical world, 'common conditions are common and rare conditions are rare'. Prevalence is what defines what is common and what is not. It gives the physician some form of direction when considering what diagnosis to make when the patient tells them their symptoms.

In short, prevalence could be considered a valuable tool to doctors and other healthcare professionals. From the point of view of the patient, when explained in simple terms, prevalence could provide them with an idea and estimate as to how many other people in the world suffer from the same condition, and can provide some reassurance occasionally that they are not alone.

In the discussion forthwith, a detailed account of some of the studies that have been performed to assess the prevalence of bone spurs and their clinical features has been described. Try not to get alarmed by all the statistics – they are just meant to give you an idea of how common bone spurs are in different parts of the body!

## b. What is the prevalence of bone spurs?

There are only a few studies that look at the exact prevalence of bone spurs, with those that do only analysing a small population group or just analysing human skeletons. As bone spurs are common in osteoarthritis, it might be interesting to look at the prevalence of osteoarthritis first before diving into the individual prevalence of bone spurs in different parts of the body.

Studies have estimated that over 20 million people in the United States suffer from osteoarthritis, so it is likely that most of these will suffer from bone spurs as well (Pereira D, 2011). At least half of these will fall in the older population group as well. While osteoarthritis is generally more common in women over the age of 50, it must be remembered that there are other factors such as weight bearing and obesity that can cause bone spurs, making bone spurs common in men as well.

The prevalence of bone spurs varies depending on the location. We have already discussed the different sites in which bone spurs can be seen. To quickly recapitulate, bone spurs are commonly seen in –

1. The spine (including the neck and lower back)

2. The knee

3. The hip

4. The shoulder

5. The hands and feet

Let's take a look at some of these in a bit more detail.

## 1. The spine

The spine extends from the lower part of the head and traces down all the way to the coccyx bone (tail bone). It includes the neck spine and the part of the spine that supports the torso. The lumbar spine is subject to constant stress due to the fact that it holds the body upright and bears the brunt of the different forces the body experiences when performing different activities.

Recently, a very interesting study reported the findings of bone spurs in pre-modern Korean skeletons that the researchers obtained from Josean tombs. They found that even these skeletons possessed a number of bone spurs, making this a condition that has been prevalent for generations! (Kim DK, 2012)

In a study assessing patients over the age of 50 in the United Kingdom, 84% of 499 men and 74% of 681 women demonstrated the presence of one or more bone spurs along their spine. Interestingly, and as expected, these bone spurs were more common in areas of the spine on which maximum stress was being placed. The majority of the patients who did have bone spurs were either older, had a higher body weight or performed regular strenuous activity that placed a lot of stress on the back. The bone spurs also caused pain in the lower back for many of the male subjects (O'Neill TW, 1999).

It is important to bear in mind that prevalence will vary amongst different study groups, and many of the studies that are performed only analyse a small group of people.

## 2. The knee

There have been a few studies that have looked at the presence of bone spurs in the knee. In one such study that conducted MRI studies on the knees of 29 patients, 15% of them had bone spurs within the centre of the knee joint. These patients were amongst the older ones in the group and they also had a higher body weight (both of which are risk factors for developing bone spurs) (Thomas R. McCauley, 2001). Other studies have shown similar results, particularly with regards to bone spurs and changes in the knee seen with osteoarthritis being more prevalent as the patient groups studied get older.

In the knee joint, ultrasound studies have shown bone spurs to be most commonly present within the joint space connecting the femur and the tibia. In more advanced cases, the joint capsule itself can be destroyed by the bone spurs and degenerative changes.

## 3. The hip

The stability of the hip joint is essential to maintain a normal degree of mobility. In osteoarthritis, changes in the hip joint can result in reduced movement and a great degree of pain. Within the United States, around 5% of the population over the age of 65 years suffer from osteoarthritis of the hip (Lane, 2007). This would imply that the same number would likely suffer from bone spurs as well. This number will only be likely to increase in the next 20 years given the rising number of the ageing population, along with the increasing number of people suffering from obesity. This would indicate that hip osteoarthritis and bone spurs will continue to be a common medical problem that will affect millions of people all over the world.

## 4. The shoulder

The shoulder joint is under constant stress, even when performing daily activities. One of the major studies performed to assess the prevalence of bone spurs in the shoulder was performed in human skeletons. Here, the researchers looked at 346 skeletons and analysed the shoulder bones and joints to look for bone spurs. They found that 28.9% of the skeletons had bone spurs around the shoulder joint area, with a majority of them occurring on the right side compared to the left (Mahakkanukrauh P, 2003). This would be consistent with the fact that most people in the world are right handed and are therefore putting their right shoulders under more stress when compared to the left.

Studies have also looked at joint degeneration in sports persons. However, not many of these actually look at how common the presence of bone spurs is, but in fact looks at whether joint degeneration occurs. We have discussed later how joint degeneration can result in the formation of bone spurs. For example, in tennis players, studies have unsurprisingly revealed that 1 in 3 of the regular or elite players have changes within their joints, suggestive of joint degeneration and tissue breakdown, placing them at risk of developing bone spurs (Maquirriain J, 2006 ).

## 5. The hands and feet

The presence of bone spurs in the hands and feet is one of the most common features seen in osteoarthritis. In particular, the formation of bone spurs in the joints of the fingers in the hand is called 'Heberdens' and 'Bouchards' nodes. Most of the studies that have actually assessed how prevalent these nodes are in patients are in fact rather old. This would probably be because as a common condition, prevalence studies that are conducted are more related to osteoarthritis than to its individual clinical findings.

Whatever the case may be, studies have consistently shown hand and feet involvement in osteoarthritis. In one such study, 7 out of 10 women over the age of 80 demonstrated the presence of bone spurs in the joints of their fingers (RL, 2007). It appears that in patients in whom arthritic changes in the hand are inherited (see genetic transmission later), osteophytes were present in all the study subjects, making it a feature that is most definitely transmitted between generations.

From the discussion above, it is clear that bone spurs are a common condition. There are a number of causes and risk factors that can affect the prevalence of this condition, and the next chapter will take a detailed look at this.

## Chapter 4 – Causes of Bone Spurs

Now that we have an understanding of the physiology behind why bone spurs occur, it is time to delve into the causes of bone spurs. In order to make things simple, we have included the causes under different subheadings.

### 1. Ageing

Unfortunately, one thing in life (other than being taxed by the government) that we cannot avoid is getting old. It brings with it a number of problems with one's health, ranging from joint pains to heart attacks and strokes. The problem is coping with these age related changes, especially if they impact on the activities of daily living.

Joint health is essential to maintain independence. Having properly functioning knees and ankles allows us to move around effortlessly and perform the activities that we so enjoy doing. With advancing age, it is normal that damage occurs to the joints and bones that are most often placed under stress.

### a. The link between ageing and osteoarthritis

We previously discussed osteoarthritis and what it means in brief. With ageing, the protective tissues that surround the joint get weaker and are more prone to breaking down and degenerating. Furthermore, the space within the joint can start to shrink as well due to loss of tissue. This change is not only seen in joints such as the knee but also the hip, shoulder and the back. Bone spurs can form as a result of this damage, and is considered by many to be one of the first signs of osteoarthritis. Bone spurs in ageing are often seen along the spine and in the feet. They are usually picked up when an x-ray is performed of the back if the patient is suffering from back pains.

## b. 'I am getting old – will I develop bone spurs?'

Getting old does not necessarily mean that you will develop bone spurs. In many cases, even if they did develop, it would not cause any symptoms and you may not even realise that you have them. Many patients who remain active do not develop bone spurs, while on the other hand patients who remain inactive can develop them. In other words, there is no way of predicting whether or not you will develop bone spurs, but there are ways you can reduce the chances of developing it, which we have discussed later.

## 2. Degenerative disease (Osteoarthritis)

Ageing is not the only cause for natural degeneration of the joints and bones in humans. Osteoarthritis, while often seen in elderly patients (primary osteoarthritis), can also be seen in younger individuals (secondary osteoarthritis). Osteoarthritis is the most common joint disease in the world with millions of people suffering from this condition. Research is being constantly conducted in this area to better understand this condition.

In the previous paragraph, we mentioned a link between ageing and osteoarthritis. Osteoarthritis often affects the weight bearing joints, which includes the spine (lower back and neck), hip and the knee. It can also affect the small joints of the hands and feet.

Osteoarthritis does not only occur with ageing. There are a number of different reasons why it can develop. These can include infections of the joints, weakness of the muscles supporting the joints, problems with metabolism and breakdown of different by-products in the body, gout and even other bone diseases.

Bone spurs can be an early sign of osteoarthritis. What this means is that bone spurs could indicate that the patient is starting to develop osteoarthritis. They may not cause any symptoms for a while, and they are usually picked up during routine investigations such as an

X-ray of the joint. Sometimes, these bone spurs can break off and enter into the joint space – these are called 'loose bodies' (sometimes called 'joint mice').

## 3. Excessive activity and stress

At work and even in sports, we can be constantly on our feet for long hours on end. Constant force and pressure can cause damage to the tissues along with tightening of the joint structures. These days, different kinds of footwear are available that will cushion the foot adequately and help minimise trauma to the under surface of the foot.

We have already discussed how sportspersons are causing constant trauma to their feet and back. Those who utilise their upper body more for their sporting activity place the joints and the bones in the arms and neck at risk of developing damage. This could, over a period of time, result in the formation of bone spurs.

In patients whose regular job involves heavy labour, lifting heavy weight and bending, repetitive and unnecessary stresses may be applied on the bones and joints, subjecting them to injury. Bone overgrowth and spur formation is therefore not uncommon in this group of people.

Women who wear high-heeled shoes will very well know the pain they can experience at the back of their heel from constant wearing of the shoes. This can place undue stress on the Achilles tendon at the point where it is attached to the heel bone, causing damage and wear and tear of the tendon and the bone. This area then becomes a site where a bone spur may develop, making wearing high-heeled shoes difficult.

## 4. Being overweight

Obesity is a common cause and risk factor for degeneration of the joints. Arthritis is often seen in patients who are overweight, and this occurs because of the constant large weight that is placed on a joint that is not designed to bear this weight. The commonly affected joints where bone spurs may be seen in obese individuals is the lower back, the knee and the foot. Of course, other joints may also be involved.

While weight related bone and joint capsule degeneration is the main cause of bone spurs in obese individuals, another reason for injury is the loss of joint stability. The constant shift in weight when walking and performing other activities can place undue stress on the bones and the joints, causing them to undergo wear and tear a lot sooner than expected for one's age. In other words, the wear and tear occurs at an earlier age in obese patients, and can limit their mobility significantly. The bone spurs can cause pain, which can further limit their activities. This can only result in the patient's weight increasing over time. This 'vicious cycle' can have a significantly negative impact on the patient's life.

Finally, obesity is also associated with high levels of certain toxins called 'adipokines'. These toxins can promote inflammation within the joint and in the body as well. By doing so, they become the fuel that ignites the process of bone spur formation.

## 5. It's in the genes...

Osteoarthritis is more common in patients who have a family history of the condition. In other words, there can be a genetic cause for developing bone spurs. This would mean that even if adequate precautions are taken to prevent arthritis and look after one's health, some people will unfortunately still develop the condition purely because another family member suffered from it.

Research has identified specific genes in certain proteins that are related to osteoarthritis, but so far no tests have been developed to identify whether a patient is at risk of developing osteoarthritis in the future.

## 6. Constant Trauma

Trauma refers to injury. In some patients, repeated injury at a site can result in the level of inflammation staying high in tissues. Let us take runners for example. It is a well-known fact that runners can suffer from a condition called plantar fasciitis. The plantar fascia is a thick band of tissue that runs across the under surface of the foot under the skin. It is attached to the heel bone at one end and the bones of the toes at the other end. It serves mainly as a shock absorber, and helps to maintain the arch of the foot. When undue and constant stress is applied to the plantar fascia, it can get inflamed and cause pain. This is called plantar fasciitis. The point at which the plantar fascia is attached to the heel bone tends to also become inflamed, and is actually very painful when pressed on. The bone tries to heal itself, and in the process can form spurs at the bottom of the heel. These are called calcaneal spurs and can be very painful.

Another site where continuous trauma can cause the development of bone spurs is the shoulder. The shoulder joint is a round joint that is protected by a group of muscles and tendons called the rotator cuff. The integrity of the rotator cuff is essential to maintain the normal function of the joint. However, in people who over-strain the rotator cuff, inflammation can occur which results from the constant rubbing of the tendons against the bones in the shoulders. This can eventually lead to the formation of bone spurs around the shoulder joint which can in turn irritate the muscles and tendons. The end effect is the patient experiencing pain when attempting to move the joint and thus a limitation in their ability to do so.

Patients who are more prone to developing shoulder injuries and bone spurs include cricket players and baseball players.

In addition to the above, bone spurs have been known to occur after suffering from a road traffic accident. During the healing process, excessive bone growth may occur at certain areas in the form of spurs and can cause pain.

## 7. Bone disease

Even though the formation of bone spurs is considered to be a part of osteoarthritis, they can also be seen following different bone diseases.

### a. Osteomyelitis

Infection of the bone is called 'osteomyelitis'. In this condition, bacteria spread through the blood into the bone and cause the infection. The disease can be rather painful and is accompanied by the patient being seriously unwell. It usually requires treatment to the hospital and a course of strong antibiotics. During the healing process, it is not uncommon for bone spurs to develop at the site of infection. These may or may not cause any problems in the future.

### b. Multiple Exostoses

Yes, this sounds extremely complex, doesn't it? To put it simply, this is a genetic condition that affects both children and adults. A detailed description on this condition is out of the scope of this book, but in short, its main feature is the presence of multiple bone spurs all over the body. The most common sites include the lower end of the thigh bone (femur) and the upper end of the bone in the lower leg (tibia). It can also be seen in the humerus bone. The bone spurs in this condition can cause a great degree of pain, especially in children and usually require removal with surgery.

## 8. Metabolic diseases

Once again, without going into too much detail regarding these, there are certain conditions where there are defects in the break down and utilisation of different proteins and substances that are essential for normal human growth. For example, some patients can develop a condition called hemochromatosis, which is where the body does not utilise iron very well. Such patients tend to develop osteoarthritis, which can in turn result in bone spur formation.

## 9. Previous surgery

If patients have undergone previous surgery to the cartilage, their chances of developing a bone spurs are higher. This is because removing the cartilage in between the bones can cause them to rub together, and the constant trauma can eventually result in osteoarthritis and bone spur formation. For example, patients who have undergone removal of the meniscus in the knee following a knee injury can develop bone spurs in that area because the knee bones rub together.

It is evident from the above discussion that there are many causes of bone spurs. When you go to see your doctor or physical therapist, they will consider all of these causes before prescribing the required treatment. It is important to bear in mind that while the above is a long list, only a few of them are common, and others are very rare. Osteoarthritis is the most common cause of bone spurs, and is likely to be the first diagnosis made. All the other causes listed eventually lead to osteoarthritis, and in effect are in fact causes of osteoarthritis themselves!

# Chapter 5 – Bone Spur Types and Clinical Features

There are a variety of bone spurs that we have discussed so far, depending on where they are located. So the question now arises – how does one know if they are suffering from a bone spur? Well, while it can be quite difficult to definitely state so from just the pain and the site of the pain, it should be considered as a possibility in all patients who suffer from the risk factors described in the previous chapter.

In this chapter, we will take a closer look at the different kinds of bone spurs based on their site, discuss the normal anatomy at first and then look through the clinical features.

## 1. Heel Spurs

Heel spurs are one of the most common types of spurs, and are seen on the under surface of the heel where the foot comes into contact with the ground. It is basically an extension of the bone as a lump of calcium that can distort the normal appearance of the heel on an x-ray. It takes a long time to develop, so it is good to know that one just does not develop heel spurs overnight – they can take months to years! Let's take a closer look at this.

### a. Normal anatomy

The heel comprises of a number of different bones, including the calcaneum (heel bone), talus, navicular bone and the small bones of the feet (metatarsals and phalanges). The calcaneum forms the site of attachment of the plantar fascia – a thick band of connective tissue that extends all the way up to the small bones of the feet. The plantar fascia bears the role of providing support to the foot by maintaining its arch and by acting as a shock absorber when walking and running.

## b. Risk factors and causes of developing heel spurs

There are many risk factors and causes that have been identified. The common ones include placing a great deal of stress on the heel from walking or running with an associated abnormal placement of the foot on the ground. Not wearing appropriate footwear to cushion the heel can also cause heel spurs. Being overweight or obese can place excess stress on the point where the plantar fascia is attached to the calcaneum, thus causing it to thicken up, get deposited with calcium and to form a bone spur.

In addition to these common reasons and risk factors, people who suffer from diabetes also seem to have a higher chance of developing heel spurs.

Other factors responsible for formation of heel spurs include overpronation of your foot (also known as flattening of foot arch), and having tight calf muscles.

## c. Symptoms and signs

Just for the purpose of clarity, symptoms refer to what a patient is experiencing, while signs are what a doctor or treating healthcare professional look for when attempting to make a diagnosis.

The most common symptom of heel spurs is pain. Many a time though patients may have heel spurs and not have any symptoms for years! When pain does occur, patients find that it only occurs when stress or weight is placed on the heel. This is because this stress can result in the onset of inflammation at the site due to constant irritation.

The pain that patients describe typically in casualty or when they see a doctor is one of a 'nail being driven into the heel'. The pain is worse in the morning after a good night's rest. This is because the plantar fascia has had time to relax at night, but during that process of relaxation can get tightened up further. So when the patient places their foot on the ground in the morning, it can stretch the tight fascia, and can thus place strains upon the heel spur. As the day progresses, the pain usually gets better and patients find that they can move around a lot easier. However, standing for long hours or going for long walks or a run can worsen the pain due to the pressure on the spur.

Doctors may be able to elicit signs that are suggestive of heel spurs or plantar fasciitis by pressing on the calcaneum to reproduce the pain. There do not need to be any specific signs other than this stimulation of pain that can be used as a bedside test to diagnose this condition.

Actually the cause of the pain is not the heel spurs itself but the soft tissue injury associated with it (inflammation of plantar fasciitis). Plantar fascia is a big strong ligament on the bottom of the foot. It stretches from the bottom of the heel bone to the ball of the foot. Over a period of time, heel spurs develop where this ligament tugs and pulls at the heel bone. This damage to the fascia can be caused suddenly (by jogging, running or dancing) or gradually (due to wear and tear of the tissues that make up plantar fascia). As plantar fasciitis and heel pain are associated with each other, chronic plantar fasciitis is also known as 'heel spur syndrome'.

## 2. Cervical Spine Spurs

Cervical spine bone spurs are not very common, but do occur. Bone spurs are a characteristic feature of several spinal diseases, including diffuse idiopathic skeletal hyperostosis (in which bone spurs are formed on the spinal ligaments), spondylosis (bone spurs cause bones in the neck or lower back to degenerate) and spinal stenosis (bone spurs result in spinal narrowing).

Cervical or neck traction is an effective treatment for cervical bone spurs. Cervical traction will reduce the pressure on spinal nerves or nerve roots. Here we take a closer look at his.

## a. Normal anatomy

The cervical spine consists of 8 vertebrae that are perfectly aligned to allow for smooth movements in a number of directions. Each vertebra has a body that forms the main part, along with the bony canal through which the spinal column runs. At the back of the vertebra is the spinous process which is what one would feel if they were to run their fingers along the lower part of the back of their neck.

In between each of the cervical vertebra are ligaments that attach the vertebrae to each other. They allow for normal movement and also maintain the alignment of the spine. Between the bodies of each vertebra is a soft intervertebral disc that cushions the bones and act as shock absorbers. Both the ligaments and the discs are under constant stress during different movements and activities.

Inflammation of the ligaments can occur when they get damaged or inflamed from different traumas. When this trauma persists for long periods of time, areas where the bone and ligaments are damaged become deposited with calcium. In addition, new bone formation occurs at the site, and this new bone and calcium deposition is what constitutes a bone spur.

Studies have shown that cervical bone spurs are seen in around 20-30% of the elderly population (Bone RC, 1974).

## b. Causes and risk factors of cervical spine bone spur formation

The most common reason why cervical spine bone spurs develop is age related osteoarthritis. With advancing age, it is natural to lose some amount of bone tissue from years and years of neck movements. In addition, the cartilage around the bones and the intervertebral discs also undergo degenerative changes.

In addition to this, recovery of tissue in the neck following some form of trauma can increase the chances of developing a bone spur. Poor neck posture places the bones and joints under a variety of stresses that can be a risk factor for the development of bone spurs.

Certain injuries such as whiplash and compression fractures can hasten the degeneration of joints, and thereby lead to the formation of bone spurs. Other conditions such as decreased blood supply, chronic illness, infection or a diminished immune system can also lead to degradation of joints in spinal column and formation of bone spurs.

We have previously mentioned diseases of the bone itself (multiple exostoses) as a cause for bone spurs. This is true with regards to the neck as well, as it is a recognised cause of multiple bone spurs in the cervical spine.

## c. Symptoms and signs

The symptoms that patients experience are similar to what they would have if there were bone spurs elsewhere in the body. In other words, in most cases, they do not cause pain by their presence alone, but do so when they press on nearby structures. Remember that the spinal cord in encased within the vertebral bones, so the bone spurs can compress on the spinal cord or the nerves that arise from it causing pain in the neck or tingling pains in the arms. Patients may have difficulty moving their neck – this is called neck stiffness. If the cervical bone spurs grow up to the extent that they impinge upon nerves or other structures, they many cause some serious effects also. This may include radiating leg and arm pain, weakness and numbness in the extremities, severe neck or back pain, restricted movements of the lower or upper body parts, and in severe cases, disability.

In some patients, cervical spine bone spurs can cause headaches along with the neck pain. More severe cases of bone spurs can compress the nerves so much that they can block the flow of nerve signals to the arms, causing weakness of the arms. As a result, patients may have difficultly handling or grasping objects, especially if the muscles of the hand are involved.

Rare cases have reported that large bone spurs can cause difficulty swallowing and difficulty breathing. This is because the bone spurs may be large enough to compress upon the food pipe or the windpipe.

## 3. Shoulder Joint Spurs

The shoulder joint is subject to a variety of stresses, so it is no surprise that spurs can form within the joint. Here we take a closer look at this.

### a. Normal anatomy

The shoulder joint is described in medical textbooks as a 'ball and socket joint'. This is because the top end of the humerus bone is shaped like a ball, while the part of the scapula bone that it is attached to is shaped like a socket (called the glenoid cavity). Other bones attached to this joint include the clavicle (collar bone) and a part of the scapula called the acromion process. The sternum (breast bone) also forms a part of the shoulder joint as it connected to it by the clavicle.

As a result, the shoulder joint is a lot more complex than it appears to be. It in fact is composed of 3 main joints – the sternoclavicular joint (between the sternum and the clavicle), the acromioclavicular joint (between the clavicle and the scapula) and the glenohumeral joint (which is the ball and socket joint between the humerus and the scapula).

Around this complex joint are different structures that aid smooth movement of the shoulder. These include muscles, tendons and small fluid filled sacs called bursa. The fluid movement of the shoulder joint is aided by a structure called the synovium, which is the smooth cartilage lining the joint.

There are 4 main muscles that help support the shoulder joint and enable movement – these are called the rotator cuff muscles. They include the supraspinatus, infraspinatus, teres minor and subscapularis. There are other muscles as well that extend from the back into the shoulder joint to help stabilise it. But the muscles are not the only structures that help stabilise the shoulder. There are a fair few ligaments that attach the different bones together thus keeping them in place when the shoulder joint is placed under stress.

Finally, the fluid filled bursa is called the subacromial bursa as it is located below the acromion process of the scapula. It prevents the rotator cuff muscles from rubbing against the acromion process during shoulder movement.

Having had a brief overview of how complex the shoulder muscle is, and how versatile it is when it comes to movement, it is only natural that this joint undergoes a great degree of trauma when performing strenuous tasks. Bone spurs can occur within the shoulder joint, and we shall now look at what causes them.

## b. Causes and risk factors of shoulder spurs

Amongst all the causes of shoulder bone spurs, osteoarthritis still remains the most common cause. It is mostly age related, and patients who develop it may notice a 'cracking' sensation when they move the joint around. The changes that occur within the shoulder joint due to osteoarthritis include loss of joint space, erosion of the bone due to constantly rubbing against each other, decrease in the amount of fluid in the bursa and thickening of the tendon and ligaments around the joint. Due to this, there is a great degree of inflammation within the joint, which leads to formation of bone spurs in the areas where there is the most narrowing and most trauma.

Another cause of bone spurs in the shoulder is overuse. While the shoulder is a strong and versatile joint, there is only so much stress that it can take. Anything over and above it can cause injury to the shoulder. Shoulder injuries are often seen in athletes, cricket players and baseball players due to the amount of stress they place on their joint. As a result, it is natural for the protective tissue to wear off over time, causing inflammation and pain within the joint. The inflammation forms a risk factor for developing bone spurs at the site of maximum trauma.

Finally, bone spurs can also occur after shoulder surgery. Though not very common, the inflammation that accompanies the postoperative period places the patient at a risk of developing bone spurs. Of course, many patients undergo extensive physical therapy after shoulder surgery, which allows for good healing and recovery back to normal joint movements.

## c. Symptoms and signs

As is with bone spurs anywhere in the body, very often patients with bone spurs do not have any symptoms whatsoever. However, with time, the bone spur can get bigger and impinge on structures within the shoulder joint, thus irritating them. This can result in pain and discomfort of the joint. The pain is typically worse when moving the shoulder joint and is better when the patient is resting the shoulder. Patients have described the pain in a number of ways, with some stating the pain is dull in character and some stating that it is sharp. Either way, pain seems to be a predominant symptom.

In addition to pain, patients also complain of a reduction in the range of movement of the shoulder joint. This means they may find it difficult to perform tasks such as raising their arm up or moving their arm outwards. This can have an impact on people's livelihood as well. For example, painters may find it difficult to pain walls if they are suffering from bone spurs in the shoulder. This progressive loss of motion is due to decreased joint space and tightening of the joint capsule (the connective tissue that surrounds the shoulder joint to keep it stable). Abduction, external and internal turning of humerus bone is also limited due to painful shoulder bone spurs.

Due to the constant irritation of the structures within the shoulder joint by the bone spurs, it is natural that inflammation occurs. This is accompanied by swelling, so patients with shoulder bone spurs can have a swollen shoulder.

If the above symptoms are severe, prompt treatment is usually warranted.

## 4. Knee Spurs

The knee joint is under constant stress especially when a person is on their feet. It can bear a significant proportion of the body's weight and can therefore be prone to injury and wear and tear. It is therefore not uncommon for bone spurs to develop within the knee joint. Here we take a closer look at this.

## a. Normal anatomy

The knee joint consists of 3 bones and a number of ligaments. The joint is designed in a way to allow limited motion but is versatile enough to handle a variety of stresses. The knee joint consists of the lower end of the femur and the upper end of the tibia and fibula bones in the leg. Between these bones are pieces of cartilage that cushion the surfaces of the bones when they move against each other, thus preventing them from getting eroded. These pieces of cartilage are called menisci. The bones are also joined together by ligaments called collateral ligaments.

At the front of the knee is a small bone called the patella, which is what is commonly called the 'knee cap'. This bone by itself does not serve any function and is in fact a bone that is formed under the surface of the large tendon of the thigh muscles. Such bones are called sesamoid bones.

The knee joint can move in a number of directions though it does seem to be limited a fair bit. The primary movement of the knee joint is called flexion, which is a movement that brings the heel towards the buttocks. Straightening out the knee joint, also called extension, is limited, as is rotation of the knee joint.

In athletes and other sportspersons, including elderly patients, the knee may be subject to movements that are not natural to the joint, resulting in excessive stretching or even tearing of the ligaments and cartilage. Constant trauma to the joint can cause inflammation and therefore result in the formation of bone spurs.

## b. Causes and risk factors

We have already briefly discussed how unnatural movements of the knee joint can place it under excessive stress. While this can be a common cause for the development of bone spurs, it is clear from evidence that the most common cause remains age-related osteoarthritis. This causes destruction of the tissues and cartilage within the joint, thus reducing the space between the bones. With more and more destruction occurring over time, the bones start to rub against each other, causing pain and inflammation. This also causes breakdown and erosion of the bone, stimulating bone cells to try and heal the affected areas. This can result in an overgrowth of bone causing bone spurs to form.

Constant trauma to the knee can also have a similar effect, resulting in bone spur formation.

These two causes remain the primary and the important causes of bone spurs in the knee.

## c. Symptoms and signs

Bone spurs in the knee develop over years so early on the patient may not have any symptoms. However, as the bone spurs get bigger, they start to press upon structures in the knee, including nerves, muscles and the nearby bones themselves. This can cause pain on movement of the knee, especially when it is extended and flexed.

Patients can have difficulty climbing stairs, and may also have difficulty standing in a place for a while and walking long distances. One of the common symptoms that patients report is a 'cracking' sensation when they move their knees.

When examined, patients will complain of pain when the doctor attempts different movement of their knees. There is usually presence of swelling due to the extensive inflammation within the joint as well. These changes are clearly evident on examination, making it a fairly straightforward case to diagnose.

It must be borne in mind that bone spurs are a feature of osteoarthritis, and that with worsening osteoarthritis comes difficulty walking. Patients may eventually need walking aids to help lessen the weight that is placed on the knee and thus to relieve pain.

## 5. Hip joint spurs

The hip joint, like other joints, is always under a lot of stress. Here we take a closer look at bone spurs within the hip and also discuss the basic anatomy of the hip joint.

### a. Normal anatomy

The hip joint, like the shoulder joint, is a ball and socket joint. The 'ball' is formed by the top end of the femur (thigh bone) while the 'socket' is formed by the pelvic bone (hip bone). A detailed discussion on each of the bones is out of the scope of this e-book, but here we shall take a closer look at the anatomy of the joint itself.

The upper end of the femur, also called the head of the femur, is rounded and fits comfortably in the socket called the 'acetabulum'. The acetabulum itself is formed from different parts of the pelvic bone. The margins of the acetabulum are protected by a layer of cartilage called the acetabular labrum. In a way, this labrum makes the acetabular cavity deeper, allowing the head of the femur to sit snugly within it.

The femur is attached to the acetabulum through a variety of ligaments. These ligaments connect the tip of the femur to the pelvic bone, along with completely encasing it in order to keep it stable.

In addition to the above structures, the hip joint is also protected by small fluid filled pockets called bursa. Around the head of the femur and inside the acetabulum is a fibrous lining called the synovium. This protects the 2 bones from rubbing against each other, thus preventing joint destruction. The join also contains nerve fibres and numerous blood vessels.

It is natural that when the hip joint is active that the structures within it and around it are placed under a variety of different stresses. These can lead to bone spur formation.

## b. Causes and risk factors

Bone spur formation in the hip is a natural consequence of ageing. We have already discussed the exact cause for age-related changes in the joint i.e. osteoarthritis. Osteoarthritis directly affects the cartilage and the synovium around the hip joint, resulting in it thinning out and exposing the surface of the bone. This whole process can take a while, sometimes years, and the patient may have no symptoms whatsoever during this time. However, when the bare areas of the bone get larger, the rubbing against each other only gets worse. This can cause rather severe inflammation around the joint and can stimulate the bone to try to produce new bone and promote calcium deposition to replace the eroded areas. This new bone and calcium is what forms bone spurs.

The ligaments around the hip joint are also under constant stress. Be it walking, running, climbing stairs or even performing yoga, the ligaments are constantly being stretched and twisted to keep the hip stable. Inflammation ensues and this can also be a contributing factor towards bone spur formation. Ligaments can also become calcified and eventually form bone spurs.

The hip joint bears a great amount of weight as well, supporting most of the upper body weight. In people who are obese, damage to the hip joint can occur due to excessive weight bearing stress. In fact, obesity is a risk factor for osteoarthritis, and is therefore a risk for developing bone spurs too.

## c. Symptoms and signs

Patients who suffer from hip spurs complain of pain on movement of the hip. In many cases, patients may not have any symptoms whatsoever, and one day might notice a bit of pain in the hip when walking or climbing stairs that they did not have before. The joint pain is absent when the patient is resting and gets worse when some form of activity is performed. Patients typically report the absence of pain when they wake up in the morning, but worsening pain through the day.

The joint may also be stiff and as a result patients may have difficulty moving the hip joint (for example – raising the leg, bringing the knee up to the chest etc.).

When examined, the doctor will perform certain movements of the hip joint in the patients that may reproduce the pain. This can include lifting the leg off the couch, moving the leg outwards or even a few twisting movements of the hip.

So as is seen above, the symptoms are similar to bone spurs elsewhere, with pain on hip movement being the primary and most annoying symptom.

## 6. Hand and Wrist Bone spurs

Hand and wrist bone spurs are a common feature of osteoarthritis. Here we take a closer look at the anatomy of the hand and discuss the causes and symptoms of bone spurs in this area.

## a. Normal anatomy

The hand and wrist bear a complex anatomy. It is this complex anatomy that allows the hand to perform so many varieties of tasks that involve different movements.

For the purpose of simplicity, we shall cover the anatomy of the wrist first and then move on to the anatomy of the hand.

The wrist joint is composed of 2 large bones and 8 small bones. The 2 large bones are in fact the lower ends of the bones in the forearm called the radius and the ulna. The 8 small bones are called the carpal bones. These bones are joined together by small ligaments that allow for a range of movement at the wrist. In addition, a number of muscle tendons pass over this joint thus facilitating its movement as well.

The hand is composed of a number of bones, muscles, tendons, synovial sheaths and ligaments. Within the palm of the hand are larger bones called metacarpals. Within the fingers are smaller bones called the phalanges. The metacarpals are connected to the phalanges through the metacarpo-phalangeal joint. Between the phalanges are the inter-phalangeal joints. It is these inter-phalangeal joints that are the sites for the formation of bone spurs. These joints help perform intricate activities such as grasping objects or pinching.

The hand and wrist bones are not subject to weight bearing stress, but can be affected by sports and activities such as gymnastics and weight lifting. However, the number one cause for formation of bone spurs is osteoarthritis.

## b. Causes and risk factors

The cause for bone spurs in the hand and wrist bones is slightly different than bone spurs that occur elsewhere. Within the interphalangeal joints, the most common cause of bone spurs is osteoarthritis. In the medical world, these bone spurs have a name and are called Heberdens nodes and Bouchards nodes. The presence of these nodes is fairly typical of osteoarthritis and many times doctors make a diagnosis of osteoarthritis based on the presence of these nodes.

Other causes and risk factors for bone spurs in the hand and wrist are rare. Age-related changes can occur with breakdown of tissues around the joints occurring as one gets older. The breakdown and degeneration of the structures that support and protect these delicate joints in the hand can result in a great degree of inflammation and pain. As a result, patients can experience a variety of symptoms that can affect them significantly. Let's take a look at the symptoms a bit further.

## c. Symptoms

As is the case with bone spurs anywhere in the body, most patients who have bone spurs in their hands and wrist may not have any symptoms for quite a while. However, as the joint degeneration progresses and gets worse, symptoms can start appear which prompts patients to go and see a doctor. Patients may also find increasing difficulty performing finer movements with their hands such as holding a cup of tea or grasping a piece of paper. All these symptoms can point towards some form of joint abnormality.

Patients can also complain of swelling of the joints in their hands. In most cases, the swelling occurs gradually over a period of time and is not something that occurs overnight. In addition to the swelling, they complain of pain on movement of the fingers and the wrist. They can sometimes also state that the joints crack when they try to move them. This cracking sensation occurs because bone spurs form within a joint that is rather narrow and has limited space between the bones. As a result, the bone spurs rub against the bone causing the cracking sensation that can in fact be felt when moving the joints.

Another symptom that patients can complain of is stiffness of the joints especially during the early hours of the morning after overnight sleep. This can get better during the day with a bit of exercise. The pain in the joints can also be quite bad early in the morning. While early morning stiffness is primarily a feature of rheumatoid arthritis, bone spurs can also cause some degree of stiffness as has been described in this paragraph.

When examined by a doctor, certain specific features are looked for. These include swelling in the interphalangeal joints and the wrist joint. As a result of the swelling, the position in which the fingers lie when the hand is relaxed may be altered. In other words, if the hand is placed on the table with the palms facing downwards, the fingers may appear irregular and as if they are pointing either outwards or inwards rather than straightforward and in close contact the table. This is because there is destruction of the joints of the hand by osteoarthritis and the bone spurs and calcium deposition can result in them healing in an irregular manner.

The other feature that may be noticed by doctors is that the swollen joints can be rather painful to touch and also painful when the joint is moved. Performing different actions such as pinching can be rather painful and certain tests may be performed to confirm whether or not the joints are inflamed due to the presence of bone spurs and inflammation.

Depending on how severe the joint involvement is, the doctors will make a decision on how to manage this appropriately.

## 7. Elbow Joint Bone Spurs

The elbow joint consists of three main bones and can be manipulated in a number of different directions. Due to this capability it is often under stress when attempting to lift weights or anything heavy, and is subject to wear and tear over time. In this section, we shall take a close look at the elbow joint itself and how bone spurs can occur within this joint and affect patients.

## a. Normal anatomy

As was mentioned above, the elbow joint is comprised of three bones - the lower end of the humerus bone, the upper end of the radius and the upper end of the ulna. The radius and the ulna are the two bones in the forearm. If one were to look at the elbow joint closely, it is evident that these three bones fit together perfectly. The radius has a nice round head that fits snugly against one part of the humerus while the ulnar has a hooked upper end that winds around and fits in a small cavity at the back of the humerus. In medical terms, the joint between the ulna and the humerus is like a hinge and is aptly called a hinge joint. The radius and the ulna are also attached to each other so that they can move in perfect synchrony when complex movements are performed at the elbow.

But the elbow joint is not only made of bones. There are a number of ligaments as well that strengthen the joint and prevent it from sustaining any injury under stress. Around the joint is a large cartilage membrane that is called the joint capsule. Within the joint capsule is fluid called synovial fluid that acts like a lubricant allowing for small motion of the elbow joint. Just think of it like oil for moving machine parts. The joint capsule itself embraces a large part of the lower end of the humerus and the upper end of the radius and ulna. It is a strong structure and protects the joint during different movements.

While not necessarily a part of the joint, it is important to know that around the joint and attached in the joint are a number of different muscles that enable joint movement. These muscles have tendons that wind around the joint and even attach to it. Blood vessels and nerve fibres also run around the joint in close proximity to it.

Different movements can occur at the elbow joint. The one with the greatest range of moment is flexion of the elbow joint which is the movement performed if one wants to contract the biceps muscle.

Straightening out of the elbow joint is limited by the bone structure. Two other movements that also occur at the level of the elbow joint are called pronation and supination. In simple terms, these are the movements that occur if one would be screwing a nut using a screwdriver.

So it is clear from the discussion above that the elbow joint is a complex joint where a number of different movements can occur, some of which are rather limited in range. When placed under undue stress, damage can occur to the cartilage and the bones resulting in the formation of bone spurs.

## b. Causes and risk factors

Osteoarthritis still remains the most common cause of bone spurs in the elbow joint. Advancing age is also a factor and osteoarthritis is closely associated with this. The gentle way that bone spurs develop within the joint remains the same, as is the case with other joints. Overuse of the joint along with degenerative changes as one gets older results in wear and tear of the cartilage and a reduction in the amount of synovial fluid between the bones. As has been mentioned previously, this synovial fluid is like oil in a machine and allows for smooth movement of the elbow joint. The cartilage that lines the bones also starts to thin out and exposes the bone surface. Due to this, the three bones start to rub against each other causing inflammation and resulting in the formation of bone spurs.

Another cause for bone spurs within the elbow joint is trauma. Sometimes, falls directly onto the elbow joint can cause fracture of either of the bones. The healing process is characterised by a great degree of inflammation and this inflammation can stimulate the formation of bone spurs again.

Overuse of the elbow joint as is the case with some athletes can also cause significant amount of injury to the joint and its cartilage. This again is a risk factor for developing bone spurs.

## c. Symptoms and signs

Many patients who suffer from bone spurs in the elbow joint do not necessarily have any symptoms. However with time, the bone spurs can get larger and can start to press upon nearby structures such as muscle tendons or even nerve fibres. This can irritate these structures to a point where patients can experience a great deal of pain when moving the elbow joint. This is the most common complaint that patients have when they go to see their doctor.

Patients may also have swelling around the elbow joint and sometimes an accumulation of small amount of fluid, which is a result of inflammation.

Upon examination of the elbow joint, there is restricted movement due to pain. In other words, when the doctor attempts to move the patients elbow joint in different directions, the patient can experience pain, which indicates the likelihood of there being some degree of inflammation, and possibly bone spurs. Sometimes, the bone spurs can even break off and float within the joint causing pain by compressing nearby structures. The joint may be swollen as well and will be tender to touch.

In rare cases, the broken of bone spur can result in a 'locked' elbow joint meaning the patient will be unable to bend or extend the elbow beyond a particular point due to pain.

It is clear from this discussion that pain is the most common symptom that patients experience when they have bone spurs in the elbow joint.

## 8. Thoracic bone spurs

### a. Normal Anatomy

Thoracic bone spurs refer to bone spurs within the vertebrae that form part of the thoracic cage. The thoracic cage refers to a number of different structures that join together and protect the lungs, heart and other various organs. Towards the front of the thoracic cage is the breastbone, which is also called the sternum. Attached to the sternum are a number of ribs that encircle the organs and eventually attach to the vertebra of the back. In total there are 12 thoracic vertebrae.

The structure of the vertebral bones is similar to those that are seen in the neck. To recap, each vertebra is composed of a body, a protruding spinous process (which is what is felt when running a finger along the back) and the pedicles. Within the vertebra lies the spinal-cord which gives off a number of nerve fibres that supply the muscles, skin and organs. Between the vertebrae lie the soft intervertebral discs which act as a cushion between the vertebrae. In other words, these intervertebral discs are shock absorbers and in a way protect the vertebral bones. Alongside the body of the vertebral bones lie a number of ligaments that align the vertebra and maintain the contour of the back.

The thoracic vertebrae are subject to a variety of stresses that range from twists and turns to bending forwards and backwards. They also bear a significant underweight especially during heavy activity. It is therefore no surprise that the thoracic vertebral bones can in fact be subject to injury and therefore form bone spurs. But it must be borne in mind that the thoracic vertebra are in fact arranged in a very stable manner and are less likely to be subject to a great deal of wear and tear and injury.

## b. Causes and risk factors

The most common cause of bone spurs in the thoracic vertebra is a natural wear and tear that occurs with ageing and osteoarthritis. The actual phenomenon itself is similar to how osteoarthritis develops in other parts of the body. While the vertebra in the lower back are usually more commonly affected by osteoarthritis, the thoracic vertebrae are not necessarily spared, though the condition is actually quite rare.

Osteoarthritis can destroy the surface of the vertebral bone and also reduce the size of the intervertebral discs. As a result, the space between the bones is reduced and the friction between the bones is increased. By rubbing against each other, the bone surfaces can become raw and inflamed, stimulating calcium and new bone formation. This new bone is what the bone spurs are. They can sometimes get large enough to cause compression on the nearby structures.

Another cause of bone spurs in the back can be injury to the back such as a fall or from a road traffic accident. During the healing process, abnormal bone may be formed which is what appears to be bone spurs on x-ray.

## c. Symptoms and signs

Patients who suffer from bone spurs in the thoracic vertebrae usually complain of pain, which is worse on movement of the back. Due to the pain, patients may have difficulty performing certain daily tasks such as bending down to pick up something from the floor or even turning around when somebody calls their name.

Sometimes bone spurs can become large enough to compress on any nerve fibres that emerge from the spinal cord or directly on the spinal cord itself. This can cause altered sensation in the areas that are supplied by the nerves, which patients usually experience as a tingling sensation or numbness.

There are a number of different nerve fibres that arise at different levels from the thoracic vertebra. For example, the nerves that arise in the level of the first thoracic vertebra supply one part of the body while those that arise from the sixth thoracic vertebra supply another part of the body. This would mean that symptoms that patients have can indicate where the bone spurs might be.

The other symptoms that patients may experience from thoracic bone spurs are fairly rare. Infections may occur in some patients and when they do, patients run a high fever and can feel extremely unwell. If the bone spurs are large enough to compress upon the main spinal cord, they may cause paralysis. Once again, this is fairly rare as bone spurs rarely become that large.

Upon clinical examination, doctors will be able to locate where the bone spurs are based on the history, clinical symptoms and signs. Patients may have tenderness when the doctor presses on the area where there are bone spurs present. Pain may be also reproduced when the doctor tries to move the patient's torso in different directions. Many times however clinical examination may be normal and bone spurs are only diagnosed after performing a few tests.

It is clearly evident in this chapter that bone spurs can occur in many parts of the body. Our body is designed in a way that it is capable of managing a variety of stresses and movements. Unfortunately, age can get in the way and wear and tear becomes a natural phenomenon. Osteoarthritis sets in, can destroy the joints and form bone spurs that are large enough to cause distressing symptoms that can affect the patient's quality of life. Early diagnosis by a physician can help control the pain and may even prevent the bone spurs from getting any larger.

In the next chapter, we shall take a look at how bone spurs are diagnosed, what investigations may be performed and what to expect when you see a doctor.

# Chapter 6 – Diagnosis of Bone Spurs

Having discussed the physiology behind how bone spurs develop, the normal anatomy of the human body and the symptoms and signs that patients experience when suffering from bone spurs, it is now time to look at how this condition can be diagnosed accurately.

If you suffer from bone spurs and do not know it yet, your visit to the doctor could be broadly divided into a number of aspects that will aid the doctor to make a diagnosis. This can include a detailed history, a clinical examination, diagnostic tests and other specialist investigations.

## 1. Clinical History

We have already looked at the history that patients present with when they see a doctor. History refers to what symptoms the patient has been experiencing and the doctor may ask a number of questions pertaining to the history. Some of the common questions that may be asked include

a. How long have you had the pain for?

b. What makes the pain worse and what makes it better?

c. Have you suffered from any injury or form of trauma recently?

d. Have you had a fever or lost any weight?

e. Do you have a family history of bone problems?

These are only a few questions that may be asked. Many a time, the questions may seem irrelevant but they are always asked in order to rule out any other serious problems. For example, in the questions above, question number four asks if the patient has had a fever or lost any weight. This is because back pain can occur due to an infection around the spinal cord such as an abscess or even tuberculosis. Weight loss can be a feature of patients who have cancer that has spread to the bone. It is important not to panic on hearing these questions as they are standard history taking methods that allow the doctor to make a definite diagnosis.

A detailed history can take anywhere between 10 to 20 minutes to conduct. Of course, depending on what the doctor thinks the likely diagnosis is from the history, the interview may be a bit longer. History taking is either conducted in a clinic setting or in a hospital ward. Remember that any information that is given to the doctor will be kept confidential and it is important to be open and honest about your symptoms so that the doctors can help you to the best of their abilities.

## 2. Clinical Examination

After a history is taken, a clinical examination is performed. It is your right as a patient to ask for a chaperone to be present if the doctor does not offer you one. Clinical examinations can vary depending upon where the doctor thinks the bone spurs might be. Furthermore, clinical examinations may be extended in order to rule out other clinical conditions that may be causing pain.

Let's take a look at this further.

A general examination is conducted for all patients seen by a doctor. These include the height, weight and body mass index. In addition, the pulse rate, blood pressure, blood glucose levels, oxygen levels in the blood and the rate of breathing may also be recorded. While these may seem irrelevant, they can in fact be markers of a more sinister process that may be undergoing within the body. For example, a fast heart rate and low blood pressure can indicate an underlying infection. In patients who have thoracic bone spurs that are compressing on the nerves and causing pain, patients may have fairly shallow breathing because they find it difficult to take in too much air due to the pain. These observations that are made by the doctors are essential for them to reach an accurate clinical diagnosis.

Further examination depends on where exactly the patient is experiencing pain. For example, patients who suffer from bone spurs in their hand may be asked to perform simple manoeuvres such as grasping the doctor's finger or lifting up a piece of paper from the table. This test helps the doctor ascertain the level of functioning the joints have along with making an estimate of how bad the damage to the joints is. The swelling of the joints and degree of pain also indicates how bad the bone spurs are and what treatment options need to be offered to the patient.

While this is only an example, the clinical signs and symptoms related to each area where bone spurs may occur has been discussed in detail in the previous chapter. Once a clinical diagnosis is made, it is investigations that usually help confirm the diagnosis.

## 3. Investigations

There are many different investigations that may be performed in order to diagnose bone spurs. These can range from simple blood tests to x-rays of specific regions and even more advanced scans. Most of these tests are performed in patients who have osteoarthritis and are struggling with pain.

Let's take a close look at some of the common investigations that may be performed if you are suffering from bone spurs.

## a. Blood Tests

Blood tests are performed in almost all patients who see a doctor. The only difference between each patient is that the specific tests requested can be different depending on what the clinical diagnosis is. In other words, if one patient were to have one set of blood tests, another patient may have a completely different set of blood tests even if they had the same condition but had a different reason for the condition occurring in the first place.

*How the blood tests are performed*

Blood tests are usually performed either in the outpatient department or when admitted to hospital. The tests take no more than a few minutes to complete. A small vein is identified and the skin over the vein in cleaned with an antiseptic solution. A sterile needle attached to a syringe is inserted into the vein and the required amount of blood is drawn. The blood sample is collected in specific bottles and is sent to the laboratory for examination.

*What are the specific tests performed?*

There are no specific blood tests for bone spurs themselves. A complete blood count (CBC) may be performed to measure the amount of haemoglobin and white blood cells in the blood. This will point out whether the patient is suffering from anemia or whether they have an infection in their body. This is important in elderly patients as low haemoglobin and an infection can be a cause of falls, and can lead to bone fractures that form bone spurs when they heal.

Another blood test that may be performed is the level of certain minerals in the blood. These include calcium and phosphate levels. Levels of calcium and phosphate are altered in patients who have osteoarthritis.

Other regular tests performed include kidney function tests and liver function tests.

In a few cases, certain specialised blood tests looking for antibodies in the blood may performed.

It is important to note that blood test results can be completely normal as well.

*How long does it take for blood test results to come back?*

The commonly performed blood tests can take a few hours to come back. If any special blood tests are performed, they can take a few days. Either way, if any results are grossly abnormal, you can be reassured that the necessary action will be taken swiftly.

## b. Joint fluid analysis

In patients in whom bone spurs have occurred due to osteoarthritis or joint disease, taking a small amount of joint fluid out may help reach a diagnosis as to the cause of the bone spurs. However, this test may not be necessary in many cases, but it is good to have an idea as to what the test involves should you have to get it done.

*What is joint fluid analysis?*

This is a procedure where a trained physician will take a small sample of fluid from the space within the joint. This is then sent to the laboratory for analysis. The procedure is performed when there is swelling within the joint or if there is a suspicion of an infection. This test is not essential to make a diagnosis of bone spurs, but can identify a cause for it so that the right treatment can be offered to the patient.

*How is joint fluid analysis performed?*

The procedure is fairly straightforward. The joint is analysed closely to identify a spot where the fluid can be obtained. The skin over the joint is cleaned with an antiseptic solution, and a small amount of local anaesthetic is injected into the skin and surrounding structures to numb the area. Once the anaesthetic agent has kicked in, a needle is inserted into the joint and the required amount of fluid is withdrawn for analysis.

*How long does the procedure take?*

Depending on which joint is aspirated to obtain fluid, the procedure can take a variable amount of time. It ranges from anywhere between 10 to 30 minutes.

*What does joint fluid analysis show?*

Well, the results of a joint fluid analysis can be completely normal. However, if there is an infection, certain cells may be present in high numbers. In osteoarthritis, there is inflammation within the joint (which is the cause for bone spurs) and the fluid may show high levels of inflammatory markers such as C-reactive protein (CRP).

*Are there any risks?*

As with any procedure, there are a few risks. The common ones include mild pain at the site where the joint is injected. Infection can occur but this is rare as the procedure is performed under complete asepsis. Bleeding into the joint can occur, but this is more common in patients who are taking blood-thinning medication such as aspirin or Warfarin. It is for this reason that joint injections are avoided in patients who are taking these medications.

## c. X-ray

An x-ray of the joint or bone where bone spurs are expected is probably the best test available to make a diagnosis. This is because bone spurs are clearly visible as small, irregular fragments of bone that are present very close to the normal bone. The test is simple to perform and is painless.

*How is an x-ray test performed?*

X-rays are performed in a diagnostic centre or within a hospital. The affected joint is exposed to x-rays and the image is projected onto and captured by a film. This is then examined by a doctor. It is a simple procedure that is absolutely painless.

*How long does it take?*

Most x-rays only take a few minutes to perform. The actual exposure to radiation is no more than a few seconds as this is sufficient to get a good enough image of the joint.

*What will the X-ray show?*

Bone spurs appear like small pieces or fragments of bone close to the bone and ligaments where bone erosion has occurred due to age-related changes or trauma. In addition to this, there may be certain other changes that doctors will look for to identify damage to the joint such as irregular bone surface, narrowed joint space or a change in the normal structure of the bone. Not every patient will have these changes, and in some patients the bone spurs may be too tiny to be seen on x-ray.

*Are there any risks?*

An x-ray test exposes the body to radiation, but the amount of radiation is so small that it is unlikely to cause any problems. Other than that, there are no other serious side effects that should concern you as a patient.

Be reassured that x-rays are tests that are performed in hundreds to thousands of patients every day. It is a completely safe test that provides useful information, especially when it comes to diagnosing bone spurs.

## d. Magnetic Resonance Imaging (MRI)

This is a specialised test that may or may not be performed as it does not necessarily provide any more information than an x-ray does. The main advantage is that the clarity of certain images seen on MRI is a lot better than an x-ray; in particular it shows the joint surfaces a lot better.

The test is avoided in patients who have metal work from a previous operation anywhere in the body. Furthermore, it costs a lot more than a simple x-ray, and given that is provides almost the same information that an x-ray does, it may not need to be performed.

## e. Bone scans

This test is rarely performed and is not necessary to make a diagnosis of bone spurs. The test can pick up any changes in the joints of the hands early on if they are affected by osteoarthritis. Bone spurs are not typically seen early in osteoarthritis, so is unlikely to show on a bone scan.

These are the common tests that are performed in diagnosing bone spurs. Of the available tests, an x-ray of the joints is the best test to make a diagnosis of bone spurs.

# Chapter 7 – Treatment of bone spurs

So far, we have covered the types of bone spurs, how common it is and how they can be diagnosed. Now we come to the interesting bit - the treatment.

Treatment of bone spurs primarily depends upon the cause. Even though treatment options vary, the aims of the treatments still remain the same. These include pain relief, reduction of inflammation, treating the cause, improving mobility and reducing the size of the bone spur. As a patient, pain is the predominant symptom that is always extremely distressing and troublesome. Patients usually seek treatment because of this pain.

*Is treatment actually necessary?*

Patients often try to just manage the pain at home as they may be rather apprehensive about seeing a doctor. Home remedies are useful and do take the edge off the pain but they do not necessarily treat the root cause. But bone spurs can have unexpected complications sometimes. This depends primarily on where the bone spurs are located and how big they are. For example, a bone spur in the heel only causes pain when walking or after standing for a prolonged period of time. On the other hand, a bone spur in the thoracic spine of the lower back can be large enough to compress on a nerve fibre or on the spinal cord and cause tingling, numbness and even loss of muscle strength and paralysis. Of course these complications are rare but must be borne in mind.

*When should I seek treatment?*

Most cases of bone spurs have no symptoms whatsoever. They may be too small to impinge on any nearby structures to cause pain. Furthermore, the inflammation levels may be too low to actually cause any symptoms. Some of the reasons to see your health care provider about a bone spur are- when you notice any abnormal growth, or you experience pain associated with the growth or there is difficulty in walking because of the pain in the heel or knees.

If you notice pain in any of the areas mentioned in the discussion previously where bone spurs may occur, it is wise to start taking some painkillers and visiting a doctor. There is no need to feel like a burden when you go to see a doctor with these complaints as it is their duty to listen to you and offer you treatment and advice.

Many patients often decide not to have any treatment as they just do not like taking any tablets. As you'll see in the forthcoming discussion, tablets are not all that is offered by a doctor to treat bone spurs. Medical and surgical treatments have advanced significantly over the last decade or two and have successfully helped patients get over the pain and inflammation that accompanies bone spurs. Unfortunately, no cure has been found yet as most of the time bone spurs are age related.

In a nutshell, if you are suffering from pain on movement of any part of the body, it is recommended that you see a physician and seek treatment.

*What are the treatment options available?*

Broadly classified, treatments can be divided into home remedies, medical treatments and even surgical treatments. Alternative treatment options are also available these days though many a time their actual efficacy and benefit is questioned. Nevertheless, a detailed discussion of the different treatment options is warranted so we should take a close look at this now.

## 1. Home remedies

There are a variety of different home remedies that are available to help reduce pain and inflammation that accompanies bone spurs.

## a. Rest

Rest is probably the most important measure to reduce the pain. For example, in patients who suffer from heel spurs, walking for prolonged periods of time or even standing in one place can cause pain. It is essential that regular breaks are taken in between to help reduce the pain, allowing the patient to mobilise a bit better. It is understandable that this may not necessarily be possible especially for patients who have to walk a fair bit for their jobs (e.g postmen or beat cops). Furthermore, rest may not be a suitable option when spurs affect the vertebra and hands, especially because these are under stress during movement and even when at rest, due to the position that the bones are aligned in at that time.

Another aspect of rest as a treatment for bone spurs includes avoiding activities that can worsen the pain. For example, in patients who suffer from bone spurs in their back, the advice is to avoid lifting anything heavy as it can worsen the pain and inflammation. In athletes who have developed heel spurs due to constant trauma and injury to the foot, avoiding athletic activities for a period of time is also recommended.

The problems with taking the rest that while the pain inflammation may subside, patients may experience the same symptoms again once they get back on their feet and back to the normal daily activities.

## b. Icepack application

Icepack application at the site of the pain can help reduce inflammation and consequently reduce pain. The procedure is simple to perform and all that is required is a crushed ice pack in a clean tea towel and applied to the area. Conventional icepacks are now available to buy at the drugstore or supermarket, which can be used as well. Icepack application for 10 to 15 min three times a day is recommended.

## c. Painkillers

Painkillers are now readily available over-the-counter and are useful in managing pain fairly effectively. Simple painkillers such as paracetamol and ibuprofen effectively target pain and reduce inflammation. It is always recommended that the doctor's advice be obtained before commencing any form of treatment.

If you're suffering from pain due to bone spurs, taking paracetamol regularly at the recommended dose should be able to control the pain during the initial stages. If despite taking paracetamol the pain continues, stronger painkillers such as non-steroidal anti-inflammatory drugs may be required. These drugs include ibuprofen and diclofenac. These medications should be taken after food as they tend to irritate the lining of the stomach and can cause gastritis. It is essential that you familiarise yourself with the information leaflet that accompanies these tablets and always seek medical advice before taking these medications.

## d. Weight loss

Obesity is a well-known risk factor for causing stress and strain to the ligaments, bones and joints in the body. In the previous chapters, we have taken a detailed look into how obesity can cause bone spurs. Given this, there is no doubt that reducing weight can reduce the chance of the bone spurs getting worse and can even prevent bone spurs from occurring in the first place.

Losing weight should not be done in an unhealthy manner. By this we mean that just stopping eating when trying to lose weight rapidly can actually be harmful to the body. If losing weight is what is required to treat bone spurs, then it should be done in a healthy manner with set goals in mind. Talk to your doctor before you go on a weight-loss plan. Seek the help of a dietician if required. They can offer you invaluable advice on what to eat and what not to eat which can help you lose weight healthily by only shedding body fat and maintaining muscle mass.

Try a diet of healthy fruit and vegetables and lean meat. In the United Kingdom, it is now recommended that every person eat at least five portions of fruit and veg a day. Avoid fried foods, bread, rice and other foods that are high in sugar such as cookies and chocolates.

Bone spurs should not stop the patient from performing exercise. Remember that weight-loss exercise can be performed without putting any stress on the joints when bone spurs are present. For example, in patients who suffer from heel spurs and who are unable to go for long walks or a jog, exercises such as swimming and cycling can provide the same benefits of losing fat and subsequently losing weight. It is important to continue to observe a healthy diet while performing an exercise routine to lose weight.

Once the patient has lost weight, the stress that is placed on the bones and joints is significantly reduced. Patients may even find that the pain they experienced previously is now better. But just because the pain is better and you have lost weight, it does not mean that the diet and exercise plan should be abandoned. Continuing the plan as you were and this will promote a healthy lifestyle and a long and happy life.

## e. Specific home remedies

This section refers to specific cases of bone spurs affecting different parts of the body. For example, patients who suffer from heel spurs should wear proper footwear that is comfortable and adequately cushioned to protect the heel from trauma or injury when walking or running. These days, custom-made footwear and insoles are available to help cushion the foot and reduce pain.

In patients with thoracic and lower back bone spurs, it is essential that they keep an erect and normal posture when sitting or standing. These days, ergonomic chairs are available which are designed to mould to the contours of the body, supporting each part of the back adequately. This is recommended in people who sit at a desk for long hours as a part of their job.

Most employers now have health and safety regulations for employees who will spend long hours by the desk. While this may seem to be in the interests of the employers themselves to prevent litigation, following the recommendations has a number of benefits in reducing the amount of stress on the neck and back. While age-related changes cannot be avoided and bone spurs may still occur due to this, the additional trauma that can be experienced from abnormal posture that results in pain can be avoided by just a few simple measures.

These are some of the common home remedies that are recommended for managing patients with bone spurs. As is clearly evident, these do not form a cure in any sense would only allow patients to get over their pain and continue with their normal activities.

## f. Natural remedies

Herbs have been used for centuries for treating various ailments. Several herbal remedies help in blocking the pain messages and relieving pain. Although herbal remedies are natural and safe, it is advisable to consult your physician before you start any herbal remedy.

Although there is not a lot of clinical evidence to support many of the claims of natural remedies, it is widely believed that herbal remedies have several beneficial properties that can relieve painful symptoms associated with bone spurs. Some of the natural remedies that can help you alleviate the symptoms include chamomile, curcumin, capsaicin, flaxseed, apple cider vinegar and bromelain. All these ingredients possess natural anti-inflammatory properties that provide relief from pain and inflammation associated with bone spurs.

Capsaicin is available in the form of topical application. You need to apply this cream four to five times in a day as it provides only temporary relief. Turmeric is an effective natural remedy for bone spur pain. The active ingredient in turmeric is curcumin, which possesses anti-inflammatory properties. Consume 500 to 1000 mg of curcumin on an empty stomach daily, preferably in the morning. You can massage the affected part with a cloth dipped in warm linseed oil. Wrap it with another cloth to keep the area warm. Chamomile tea, rose hip and horsetail consist of therapeutic properties that accelerate the healing process of bone spurs.

Apple cider vinegar is another natural remedy that helps in relieving the pain of bone spur. Soak the affected area in apple cider vinegar for as much of the day as possible.

Adding sodium in your diet also assists in breaking down calcium so that it can be reabsorbed in to the blood. If you are on a low sodium diet for health reasons, talk to your doctor before increasing the sodium in your diet.

## g. Vitamins and minerals

Studies have found that certain vitamins promote bone health and help heal bone spurs. Vitamin D and K prevent the abnormal growth of bones. You can obtain these two vitamins from dietary sources, fortified foods and supplements. Vitamin K can be obtained from hard cheese like gouda, probiotic fermented and cultured veggies and drinks.

## h. Education

While this cannot be particularly classed as a home remedy, it is important to recognise that being aware of what bone spurs are and how they can be treated and prevented can in fact help patients manage the condition better and prevent it from getting worse in the future. One of the reasons why this guide was written was for this very purpose. Understanding the condition can help you recognise what triggers the pain and what you could do to prevent it. You can even appreciate and understand how protecting the joints can help prevent bones spurs.

## 2. Medical treatment

Some of the medical treatments are similar to the home remedies that patients attempt before seeing a doctor.

## a. Painkillers

We have previously discussed how over-the-counter painkillers can help patients control pain and improve movement of the areas affected by the bone spurs. Painkillers such as paracetamol and non-steroidal anti-inflammatory drugs can be prescribed by doctors as well. However, stronger painkillers can also be prescribed in patients who do not respond to these over-the-counter medications.

*Non-opioid analgesics*

There are times where painkillers called cyclo-oxygenase-2 inhibitors are used. These are drugs that inhibit an enzyme called cyclo-oxygenase that is responsible for inflammation and pain. Celecoxib is an example of this category of drugs. The effect of cyclo-oxygenase-2 inhibitors is similar to that of non-steroidal anti-inflammatory drugs. However, it bears the advantage that the side effects, such as irritation of the lining of the stomach or even formation of stomach ulcers, are a lot less common than is seen with non-steroidal anti-inflammatory drugs.

*Opioid analgesics*

Other prescription painkillers that are available are opioid analgesics. Opioids are basically given to relieve moderate to severe pain. These are morphine like drugs such as codeine, dihydrocodeine and tramadol. The advantage that these drugs have is that they are very effective in reducing pain. However, overuse of the drug can have serious side effects and patients can even become dependent on them. Codeine has the side effect of constipation and patients who are on tramadol on dihydrocodeine may become addicted to these tablets.

Always take any medication that is prescribed to you as it has been recommended by the doctor. Every patient is different and you may find that while one patient is given one dose of tramadol for bone spurs, another patient may be given a completely different dose. This is because there are a number of parameters that need to be considered before prescribing the drug that the doctor will look into to make sure that it is safe.

*Steroid injections*

Bone spurs are accompanied by a great degree of inflammation and pain within the joint. We have already discussed how reducing this inflammation can help promote joint movement and reduce pain. While most of the medication that we have listed above and discussed already can reduce inflammation to a great degree, sometimes it is just not enough. Patients can continue to experience pain that can bother them during day or night, affecting their life considerably. In such patients, the doctor may consider injecting the joint with a steroid.

Steroids are anti-inflammatory compounds that have an immediate effect on reducing inflammation and pain. The commonly used steroids for joint injections include hydrocortisone, methylprednisolone, dexamethasone and triamcinolone. The choice of steroid is dependent on the physician's experience of using them.

The joint injection procedure is similar to how it has been described when obtaining a fluid sample from the joint. To briefly recap this, the area where the bone spur is present is located through x-ray and clinical examination. The skin over the area to be injected is cleaned with an antiseptic solution and the skin and the surrounding tissues are numbed using a local anaesthetic agent. A needle attached to a syringe containing the required dose of steroids is then passed into the joint and the joint is injected with the steroid.

The steroid starts to act on the inflamed surface and reduces the pain almost immediately. It does not however get rid of the bone spur. It only reduces the inflammation of the tissues that are surrounding the bone spur and that are being irritated by it.

Once the injection is complete, the patient is absorbed for a short amount of time and discharged home. It is advised to avoid any strenuous activity that may involve the joint for a few hours. Following this the patient can get back to their normal daily routine.

Steroid injections usually take no more than 10 to 15 min to perform. The effects of the steroids can last anywhere between a few weeks to a few months. Due to this, if the pain returns, patients may require repeat injections in the future.

There are very few risks associated with steroid injections. The common ones include mild bleeding or bruising at the site of injection, pain at the site of injection and maybe some mild swelling. This will usually pass in a few hours and is nothing to worry about. The more serious risks are actually quite rare. One such risk includes that of infection but the chances of this occurring are very low as the procedure is performed in sterile conditions. Bleeding into the joint is another rare complication and is usually seen in patients who are taking blood-thinning medication such as aspirin or warfarin. It is for this reason that joint injections are avoided in patients taking these medications.

Steroid injections are also avoided in patients who may be having in infection within the joint already. In addition to this, steroids can alter blood glucose levels in patients. This means that if steroids are injected in patients who have diabetes, their blood sugar levels can go haywire, making control of their diabetes quite difficult. Steroids are therefore used with caution in these patients.

One of the reasons why steroid injections may be given to the patient is to prepare them for physical therapy and a rehabilitative program. This aspect of bone spur management has been described below.

## 3. Physical therapy

Physical therapy is another form of treatment that can be offered to patients with bone spurs. It is delivered to the patient through trained physical therapists who have great degree of experience in managing patients with bone spurs. There are a variety of treatments that can be offered as a part of physical therapy and it is not just limited to exercise as one would assume.

### The aim of physical therapy

The aim of a physical therapy program is to improve joint movement, reduce pain and enhance the quality-of-life of patients.

It is important to recognise the fact that physical therapy is in no way a cure for bone spurs. In most cases, physical therapy is targeted towards patients who suffer from heel spurs rather than bone spurs elsewhere in the body. The discussion held below will mostly pertain to the role of physical therapy in managing patients with heel spurs, but any other areas that may benefit will also be mentioned as well.

Physical therapists will advise patients to attempt a number of different home remedies as has been discussed above to help reduce pain due to bone spurs. This can include rest, icepack application and even a recommendation of steroid injections.

*Stretching*

As a patient, it may be hard to believe that stretching is in fact a treatment for bone spurs but it appears that by itself it has tremendous amount of benefit in reducing pain. Of course, stretching has to be performed in a particular manner in order to reduce the pain when it comes to heel spurs, and physical therapists will offer patients a clear-cut technique and easy to perform methods that they can carry out at home.

We have already discussed how plantar fasciitis can be a risk factor for developing bone spurs. Stretching the plantar fascia can help reduce the pain that limits mobility. A simple stretch like gently pulling the toes and the upper part of the foot towards the shin can place the plantar fascia under a reasonable amount of stress, stretching it gently. Another method to stretch the plantar fascia is to stand on the edge of a step or the staircase and gently move your heel towards the ground. This stretches the plantar fascia along with the Achilles tendon and calf muscle. Performing these stretches for up to 10 to 15 min especially after waking up in the morning can help reduce the pain significantly. Further treatment sessions can be performed at any time during the day if the heel spurs are causing a problem.

Similar stretching exercises are available when bone spurs affect other parts of the body. However, a great degree of care needs to be taken especially if the bone spurs affect the cervical, thoracic and lumbar spine, as they may be very close to the spinal cord. Given this fact, stretching exercises are usually avoided. As such, it appears that stretching is probably the best form of treatment when it comes to managing bone spurs in the heel. The timeframe and success of stretching and other forms of physical therapy depends upon the ability to restore the space and proper function of the joint.

*Massage treatment*

Once again, massage therapy is a form of physical therapy that is primarily useful in managing patients with heel spurs. This is because the structures that require massaging are right under the skin in the case of heel spurs but not so in the case of spurs that are present in any other joint. Furthermore, the cause for heel spurs is inflammation of the plantar fascia that lies directly beneath the skin. On the other hand, the cause for bone spurs elsewhere is due to the destruction of the joint that lies deep under the skin and is therefore not accessible to massage therapy.

While going into great detail regarding how massage therapy is performed is out of the scope of this book, it is good to have an idea of what to expect when a physical therapist performs this procedure. The first thing to remember is that massage therapy is not like what you have seen on television where the muscles are being gently massaged. Instead, a deep tissue massage is what is offered to the patient. The aim of the treatment is to help relax the tissues and plantar fascia and improve the blood supply to the area near the bone spur. Massage therapy also helps stretch the plantar fascia and we have already discussed how beneficial this can be to the patient.

There are a number of videos that have available on YouTube that describe how massage therapy is performed to manage heel spurs. In addition to this, there are a number of different products that are now available online that can help with massage therapy and stretching.

*Massage therapy*

The deep massage produces direct heat on the calcified area, and also increases the elasticity of the adjacent tissues. This helps to dissolve calcification, a crucial step for heel spur healing. It also reduces the presence of certain substances in the blood that may generate and sustain pain and increase the release of endorphins (natural painkillers) that help in lessening the pain.

Inflammation of plantar fascia is another important cause of foot bone spurs. Deep tissue massage not only gives relief from bone spurs, but also alleviates the pain and inflammation of plantar fasciitis.

*Ultrasound therapy*

The principle behind ultrasound therapy is the delivery of deep heat to the structures that it is being delivered to. It is available and effective in patients who suffer from bone spurs in the heel. It may not necessarily be useful in treating patients who have bone spurs elsewhere.

The advantage of ultrasound therapy is the fact that it can penetrate the superficial tissues and deliver the required effect to the deeper tissues. By generating heat it can improve the blood supply to the plantar fascia and also promote relaxation of the surrounding muscles and ligaments. Any inflammation and swelling at the site as well is reduced to a great extent. All these effects combined together help reduce pain and promote patient mobility. Besides these effects, ultrasound also has a number of chemical effects such as oxidation and depolymerisation. While these terms do sound complicated, it is good to know that these effects are also helpful in reducing inflammation and pain.

Ultrasound therapy is just a temporary measure and is in no way a cure. Recurrent treatment sessions may be required to help patients overcome the pain that accompanies bone spurs. It can also be used in managing patients with bone spurs in the knee, shoulder and hip, but it is most commonly used on the heel.

It is essential that ultrasound therapy be delivered by a trained professional like a physical therapist. The reason behind this is that there may be a few side effects such as thinning of the bone (osteoporosis) and even a small amount of bleeding within the bone. These effects are rare but are identified a lot sooner if treatment is offered by a physical therapist or health care professional.

*Shortwave diathermy*

This is a specialised treatment that is useful in managing pain that arises due to bone spurs within the spine. However this application is not limited to this and it can be utilised when inflammation affects the shoulder joint, elbow joint and even the hips and the knees.

Shortwave diathermy is a high-frequency alternating current that generates heat when directed towards a structure. The heat is more deep-seated and therefore has positive effects in patients with bone spurs. Once again, it is recommended that this treatment be offered by trained professionals as there are certain limitations and certain situations where the treatment should not be given.

*Orthoses*

Orthoses refers to specific devices that can be utilised in managing pain in patients with bone spurs. These are usually custom-made and specific to each patient. Physical therapists will help design these after extensively assessing the patient's requirements.

These days, orthoses are easily available online. In most cases, they are generic in that they can be utilised by any patient. Some of the orthoses that are available are useful in managing bone spurs and plantar fasciitis. They help keep the plantar fascia stretched at night and thus help reduce the pain that patients experience early in the morning. Orthoses are also available to maintain posture and an erect spine. In patients who have large bone spurs, care needs to be taken before utilising any form of orthoses. It is essential that a doctor's advice be taken and physical therapists perform a detailed examination to make sure that this is in the best interests of the patient.

## 4. Alternative treatments

The commonly used treatments have already been described but there do exist other treatments that patients may find useful.

*Yoga*

Yoga involves a variety of postures and stretches that are both relaxing and therapeutic. In patients with bone spurs, their effect is primarily that of stretching. Yoga has shown to improve cardiovascular function meaning more blood is pumped around the body. This will include an increased blood supply to the areas where bone spurs are present. This increased blood supply helps reduce inflammation and pain. Yoga also helps to strengthen muscles and improve overall balance.

Yoga is particularly helpful in managing bone spurs that involve the spine. If you decide to take up yoga, make sure that you have the all clear from your doctor first. Following that, make sure that your yoga instructor is fully qualified and understands the various postures that you should and should not be performing. There are various bending and stretching exercises that are available to patients who decide to undertake Yoga, all of which helps strengthen the spine.

Yoga by itself only helps patients manage their symptoms better but again is not a cure for bone spurs. It does however improve a patient's mood and can improve the quality of life as well.

*Supplements*

We already mentioned above how blood tests can reveal an alteration in the levels of calcium and phosphate in the blood in patients who suffer from osteoarthritis and bone spurs. Supplements are now available that can help replenish these minerals and in turn help strengthen the bones. It is important to realise that calcium and phosphate and other minerals that are required to maintain bone health are available in foods as well. However not everyone can get the right amount and even if they do, it may be that the minerals are not being absorbed sufficiently from the ingested diet. In such cases, calcium supplements are most certainly beneficial. They are often prescribed to elderly patients today as osteoarthritis is now a well-recognised condition associated with ageing.

There are many other over-the-counter supplements available these days that claim to help improve joint strength and rejuvenate joint tissues. These natural products include evening primrose oil, glucosamine supplements and shark cartilage. These products essentially help reduce inflammation and most of the evidence that supports its use is anecdotal. This means that there are no scientific studies or large clinical trials that have confirmed their actual benefit in helping patients who suffer from bone spurs. The benefit primarily is from patient reports and you may find that the treatment may help while another patient may find that it does not.

*Chiropractic management*

Chiropractic is a branch of alternative medicine that is based on the principle that a properly aligned spine is essential to maintain health. In patients with bone spurs, chiropractic treatment appears to help reduce pain and inflammation. It also claims to slow down the degenerative process that leads to bone spurs in the first place. However, it does not offer a cure.

Chiropractic treatment should be delivered with caution in patients who have bone spurs that affect the spine. Chiropractors will be aware of this and may perform certain preliminary tests such as an x-ray to ensure that there are no bone spurs that are irritating or pressing on the spinal cord. The vertebral column is gently realigned through certain manipulations. By doing so, the blood supply and the conduction of signals through the nerves are improved significantly. This can help reduce inflammation and pain.

*Acupuncture*

Acupuncture is an age-old treatment remedy that involves the insertion of tiny needles at certain strategic points within the body so as to alleviate pain and reduce inflammation. It has been used in managing bone spurs that involve the shoulder and heel, though they can be used elsewhere as well. A detailed discussion on acupuncture techniques is out of the scope of this book but is well worth knowing that this treatment option is available if required.

The principle behind acupuncture is that by stimulating certain points in the body and certain nerve fibres, the blood supply can be enhanced and inflammation can be reduced. It is delivered by trained acupuncturists. Is important to realise that it does not offer a cure in anyway and may or may not be effective in some patients.

## 5. Surgical treatment

Sometimes, despite taking all the above measures, bone spurs can persistently cause pain to the patient. In such cases, surgical treatments may be considered.

*Can surgical treatment help?*

The aim of surgery is to remove the bone spur and thus relieve the pressure on any structures that it was compressing upon. There are a variety of procedures that are available for bone spurs that occur in different parts of the body. The question that may arise in patient's minds is whether or not the procedure is actually necessary and if it is conducted whether it is a cure. The answer to that is that surgery can help get rid of bone spurs but unfortunately they do tend to recur. The procedure is only performed if the symptoms are so bad that the patient is unable to perform any sort of activity. It is also considered if the bone spurs are compressing on the nerve fibres or even on the spinal cord.

*Surgical treatments offered*

In the case of heel spurs, surgery is performed to help release the plantar fascia from its attachment to the heel bone. By doing so, it is reduces the stress that the plantar fascia undergoes, this reducing inflammation and pain. Any bone spurs that may be present in the heel can also be removed. Following the procedure, certain basic measures need to be followed such as wearing proper footwear and even resting the foot after surgery. Of course, surgery is not without complications and patients may sometimes experience numbness in the area along with some scarring and rarely infections. The surgeon will always perform a detailed examination of the patient prior to placing them under the knife. This will help them ascertain whether or not the treatment will be helpful to the patient and whether they should undergo it in the first place.

Bone spurs that affect the vertebral column are a lot more complicated. Surgery is also a lot more complex. As we have discussed earlier, bone spurs can sometimes grow large enough to compress on the spinal cord and cause muscle weakness. So it is essential that the surgeon be careful when extracting these bone spurs. As is the case with any surgery, the benefits of performing the surgery against the risks of developing complications have to be weighed up before considering this as an option. In many cases, the benefits only outweigh the risks if the symptoms are severe enough to have a significant impact on the patient's life.

In the cases of bone spurs that affect the knee and hip, there is usually a great degree of degeneration that has affected the bones within the joint due to osteoarthritis. In such cases, bone spurs removal by itself may not be sufficient and joint replacement surgery may be required. The decision of course will be made once investigations are completed and a discussion has been held between the patient and the surgeon regarding the benefit of joint replacement.

*How is a surgical procedure performed?*

A detailed discussion on how exactly surgery is performed in patients who have bone spurs is out of the scope of this book. However the general procedure involves obtaining consent from the patient first and the utilisation of general anaesthetic. The aim is to shave off the bones rather tham to remove it completely. Surgery can take a few hours to perform depending on which part of the body is being operated on.

Patients are usually required to stay in hospital for a few days after the procedure to ensure healthy recovery. Advice will be given to the patient regarding what they can and cannot do. Physical therapy may be offered as well to help patients get back to their normal activities in a safe and effective manner. This may take a short while but it is essential that the area where the surgery has been performed heals adequately before attempting any activity. In most cases, follow-up appointments are arranged by the surgeon to review the site of surgery and once they give the go-ahead there is no reason why you should not get back to your normal daily routine.

*Are there any risks with surgery?*

Any surgical procedure has risks. They can be either due to the anaesthetic agent that is used or due to the surgery itself. Patients can take a few days to recover from surgical procedures before getting back to their normal daily activities.

Risks depend on where the procedure is performed. In the case of surgical treatment of heel spurs, patients can only experience mild symptoms such as bleeding or bruising at the site of surgery. Pain may also occur at the site. Infections are rare and so are allergic reactions to the anaesthetic agent. If they do occur be reassured that treatment is always at hand and seek medical advice if you feel you need it.

Sometimes, risks of surgery can be a lot more serious. This is usually the case with surgery that involves removal of bone spurs that are around the spine. There is risk of nerve damage during the surgery, which can cause paralysis. But it is good to remember that experts who have plenty of experience perform these procedures.

Remember, if you have any doubts, always discuss any concerns you have with your doctor. They will be more than happy to give you the information that your need and answer any questions that you have.

## 6. Prognosis

There is not a lot to discuss regarding the prognosis of bone spurs. Most cases resolve with conservative measures and only those that cause severe symptoms require surgery. Symptoms are resolved effectively through these various measures that we have already discussed, but bear in mind that these are not a cure. Even with surgery, there is a small chance that the bone spurs can recur again and may require further input.

There are no clear statistics on the long-term prognosis of bone spurs. The statistics that are available are relevant more to osteoarthritis or the disease that causes the bone spurs.

# Chapter 8 – Future Care

In this e-book, we have discussed in detail the different kinds of bone spurs, how exactly they occur and what treatment options are available. As a patient, it is good to know how to look after yourself when it comes to treating bone spurs that are already present or preventing the formation of new bone spurs.

This e-book has offered a comprehensive review of the different risk factors that are involved in the formation of bones spurs. We also looked at different home remedies that can help treat this condition. Simple steps such as losing weight and wearing well-fitted footwear can help prevent the formation of bone spurs. Of course, in some cases, osteoarthritis is inevitable as a normal part of ageing and bone spurs will occur despite taking every precaution required.

Research is ongoing in attempting to evaluate different measures that can be taken to prevent osteoarthritis. Even though plenty of papers have been published there does not seem to be anything particularly related to bone spurs alone. There is surprisingly very little research that only deals with bone spurs. This is probably because they form a small part of a spectrum of signs and symptoms that occur in various clinical conditions. There is no doubt however that at some point new treatments will be available that may help prevent bone spurs.

There are a number of places where treatment is now available to manage bone spurs. Of course, your doctor has to be your first port of call. If you're looking for devices that will help manage the pain, websites like Amazon.com now have an extensive collection of different equipment that will help patients with bone spurs. Online sales of equipment have now made life very easy for patients to purchase anything they require from the comfort of their own homes. Even gymnasiums now have physical therapists who may be able to guide you in the right direction when it comes to managing bone spurs.

Remember this – bone spurs are a natural phenomenon of ageing. Despite the symptoms that they cause, there are treatments available that can effectively help patients manage the pain and go about their normal daily activities. Life and the way you lead it should not be any different just because you suffer from bone spurs. You can enjoy the activities you love and spend time doing what you're passionate about.

We hope that you have enjoyed reading this e-book on management and treatment of bone spurs. We hope that it has provided you with some valuable information that you could use either to treat yourself or a loved one. Please note that while this e-book has offered detailed advice, it does not replace medical treatment in any way. Always seek help from your doctor if you have any concerns and before commencing any form of treatment.

# Bibliography

Bone RC, N. A. (1974). Evaluation and correction of dysphagia-producing cervical osteophytosis. *Laryngoscope* , 84:2045-2050.

Kim DK, K. M. (2012). Vertebral osteophyte of pre-modern Korean skeletons from Joseon tombs. *Anat Cell Biol* , 45(4):274-281.

Lane. (2007). Osteoarthritis of the hip. *N Engl J Med* , 357:1413-21.

Mahakkanukrauh P, S. P. (2003). Prevalence of osteophytes associated with the acromion and acromioclavicular joint. *Clinical Anatomy* , Nov;16(6):506-10.

Maquirriain J, G. J. (2006 ). Is tennis a predisposing factor for degenerative shoulder disease? A controlled study in former elite players. *Br J Sports Med* , May;40(5):447-50.

O'Neill TW, M. E. (1999). The distribution, determinants, and clinical correlates of vertebral osteophytosis: a population based survey. *The Journal Of Rheumatology* , 26(4):842-8.

Pereira D, P. B. (2011). The effect of osteoarthritis definition on prevalence and incidence estimates: a systematic review. *Osteoarthritis Cartilage* , 19(11):1270-85.

RL, U. (2007). Proximal interphalangeal joint arthrodesis using the tension band technique. *Journal of Hand Surgery* , 32:914-7.

Thomas R. McCauley, P. R.-H. (2001). Central Osteophytes in the Knee. *American Journal of Roentgenology* , 176:2,359-364.

# Index

Notes: